HOW TO GET LAID

FOR MEN

The Ultimate Guide in Your Fight for Some Action

R. J. Duncan

*I dedicate this book to everyone who strives to be better today
than they were yesterday*

HOW TO
GET LAID

For Men

R J DUNCAN

There are only a few things that can help you get laid. It isn't magical, it isn't impossible; it doesn't take much to do it. I truly believe that anyone can get laid and I hope after you've read this book, you will agree.

Turn the page to discover that one thing!

- -TAKE A SHOWER

- -GET A HAIRCUT

- -ASK HER OUT

- -OPEN WITH A JOKE

- -DON'T BE CREEPY

- -WEAR A LOVE-GLOVE

-TAKE A SHOWER

-GET A HAIRCUT

-ASK HER OUT

-OPEN WITH A JOKE

-DON'T BE CREEPY

-WEAR A LOVE-GLOVE

-TAKE A SHOWER

-GET A HAIRCUT

-ASK HER OUT

-OPEN WITH A JOKE

-DON'T BE CREEPY

-WEAR A LOVE-GLOVE

-TAKE A SHOWER

-GET A HAIRCUT

-ASK HER OUT

-OPEN WITH A JOKE

-DON'T BE CREEPY

-WEAR A LOVE-GLOVE

- -TAKE A SHOWER

- -GET A HAIRCUT

- -ASK HER OUT

- -OPEN WITH A JOKE

- -DON'T BE CREEPY

- -WEAR A LOVE-GLOVE

-TAKE A SHOWER

-GET A HAIRCUT

-ASK HER OUT

-OPEN WITH A JOKE

-DON'T BE CREEPY

-WEAR A LOVE-GLOVE

-TAKE A SHOWER

-GET A HAIRCUT

-ASK HER OUT

-OPEN WITH A JOKE

-DON'T BE CREEPY

-WEAR A LOVE-GLOVE

-TAKE A SHOWER

-GET A HAIRCUT

-ASK HER OUT

-OPEN WITH A JOKE

-DON'T BE CREEPY

-WEAR A LOVE-GLOVE

-TAKE A SHOWER

-GET A HAIRCUT

-ASK HER OUT

-OPEN WITH A JOKE

-DON'T BE CREEPY

-WEAR A LOVE-GLOVE

-TAKE A SHOWER

-GET A HAIRCUT

-ASK HER OUT

-OPEN WITH A JOKE

-DON'T BE CREEPY

-WEAR A LOVE-GLOVE

-TAKE A SHOWER

-GET A HAIRCUT

-ASK HER OUT

-OPEN WITH A JOKE

-DON'T BE CREEPY

-WEAR A LOVE-GLOVE

-TAKE A SHOWER

-GET A HAIRCUT

-ASK HER OUT

-OPEN WITH A JOKE

-DON'T BE CREEPY

-WEAR A LOVE-GLOVE

-TAKE A SHOWER

-GET A HAIRCUT

-ASK HER OUT

-OPEN WITH A JOKE

-DON'T BE CREEPY

-WEAR A LOVE-GLOVE

- TAKE A SHOWER

- GET A HAIRCUT

- ASK HER OUT

- OPEN WITH A JOKE

- DON'T BE CREEPY

- WEAR A LOVE-GLOVE

-TAKE A SHOWER

-GET A HAIRCUT

-ASK HER OUT

-OPEN WITH A JOKE

-DON'T BE CREEPY

-WEAR A LOVE-GLOVE

-TAKE A SHOWER

-GET A HAIRCUT

-ASK HER OUT

-OPEN WITH A JOKE

-DON'T BE CREEPY

-WEAR A LOVE-GLOVE

-TAKE A SHOWER

-GET A HAIRCUT

-ASK HER OUT

-OPEN WITH A JOKE

-DON'T BE CREEPY

-WEAR A LOVE-GLOVE

- -TAKE A SHOWER

- -GET A HAIRCUT

- -ASK HER OUT

- -OPEN WITH A JOKE

- -DON'T BE CREEPY

- -WEAR A LOVE-GLOVE

-TAKE A SHOWER

-GET A HAIRCUT

-ASK HER OUT

-OPEN WITH A JOKE

-DON'T BE CREEPY

-WEAR A LOVE-GLOVE

-TAKE A SHOWER

-GET A HAIRCUT

-ASK HER OUT

-OPEN WITH A JOKE

-DON'T BE CREEPY

-WEAR A LOVE-GLOVE

-TAKE A SHOWER

-GET A HAIRCUT

-ASK HER OUT

-OPEN WITH A JOKE

-DON'T BE CREEPY

-WEAR A LOVE-GLOVE

-TAKE A SHOWER

-GET A HAIRCUT

-ASK HER OUT

-OPEN WITH A JOKE

-DON'T BE CREEPY

-WEAR A LOVE-GLOVE

- -TAKE A SHOWER

- -GET A HAIRCUT

- -ASK HER OUT

- -OPEN WITH A JOKE

- -DON'T BE CREEPY

- -WEAR A LOVE-GLOVE

-TAKE A SHOWER

-GET A HAIRCUT

-ASK HER OUT

-OPEN WITH A JOKE

-DON'T BE CREEPY

-WEAR A LOVE-GLOVE

-TAKE A SHOWER

-GET A HAIRCUT

-ASK HER OUT

-OPEN WITH A JOKE

-DON'T BE CREEPY

-WEAR A LOVE-GLOVE

-TAKE A SHOWER

-GET A HAIRCUT

-ASK HER OUT

-OPEN WITH A JOKE

-DON'T BE CREEPY

-WEAR A LOVE-GLOVE

-TAKE A SHOWER

-GET A HAIRCUT

-ASK HER OUT

-OPEN WITH A JOKE

-DON'T BE CREEPY

-WEAR A LOVE-GLOVE

-TAKE A SHOWER

-GET A HAIRCUT

-ASK HER OUT

-OPEN WITH A JOKE

-DON'T BE CREEPY

-WEAR A LOVE-GLOVE

-TAKE A SHOWER

-GET A HAIRCUT

-ASK HER OUT

-OPEN WITH A JOKE

-DON'T BE CREEPY

-WEAR A LOVE-GLOVE

-TAKE A SHOWER

-GET A HAIRCUT

-ASK HER OUT

-OPEN WITH A JOKE

-DON'T BE CREEPY

-WEAR A LOVE-GLOVE

-TAKE A SHOWER

-GET A HAIRCUT

-ASK HER OUT

-OPEN WITH A JOKE

-DON'T BE CREEPY

-WEAR A LOVE-GLOVE

-TAKE A SHOWER

-GET A HAIRCUT

-ASK HER OUT

-OPEN WITH A JOKE

-DON'T BE CREEPY

-WEAR A LOVE-GLOVE

-TAKE A SHOWER

-GET A HAIRCUT

-ASK HER OUT

-OPEN WITH A JOKE

-DON'T BE CREEPY

-WEAR A LOVE-GLOVE

-TAKE A SHOWER

-GET A HAIRCUT

-ASK HER OUT

-OPEN WITH A JOKE

-DON'T BE CREEPY

-WEAR A LOVE-GLOVE

-TAKE A SHOWER

-GET A HAIRCUT

-ASK HER OUT

-OPEN WITH A JOKE

-DON'T BE CREEPY

-WEAR A LOVE-GLOVE

-TAKE A SHOWER

-GET A HAIRCUT

-ASK HER OUT

-OPEN WITH A JOKE

-DON'T BE CREEPY

-WEAR A LOVE-GLOVE

-TAKE A SHOWER

-GET A HAIRCUT

-ASK HER OUT

-OPEN WITH A JOKE

-DON'T BE CREEPY

-WEAR A LOVE-GLOVE

-TAKE A SHOWER

-GET A HAIRCUT

-ASK HER OUT

-OPEN WITH A JOKE

-DON'T BE CREEPY

-WEAR A LOVE-GLOVE

-TAKE A SHOWER

-GET A HAIRCUT

-ASK HER OUT

-OPEN WITH A JOKE

-DON'T BE CREEPY

-WEAR A LOVE-GLOVE

-TAKE A SHOWER

-GET A HAIRCUT

-ASK HER OUT

-OPEN WITH A JOKE

-DON'T BE CREEPY

-WEAR A LOVE-GLOVE

-TAKE A SHOWER

-GET A HAIRCUT

-ASK HER OUT

-OPEN WITH A JOKE

-DON'T BE CREEPY

-WEAR A LOVE-GLOVE

-TAKE A SHOWER

-GET A HAIRCUT

-ASK HER OUT

-OPEN WITH A JOKE

-DON'T BE CREEPY

-WEAR A LOVE-GLOVE

-TAKE A SHOWER

-GET A HAIRCUT

-ASK HER OUT

-OPEN WITH A JOKE

-DON'T BE CREEPY

-WEAR A LOVE-GLOVE

-TAKE A SHOWER

-GET A HAIRCUT

-ASK HER OUT

-OPEN WITH A JOKE

-DON'T BE CREEPY

-WEAR A LOVE-GLOVE

-TAKE A SHOWER

-GET A HAIRCUT

-ASK HER OUT

-OPEN WITH A JOKE

-DON'T BE CREEPY

-WEAR A LOVE-GLOVE

-TAKE A SHOWER

-GET A HAIRCUT

-ASK HER OUT

-OPEN WITH A JOKE

-DON'T BE CREEPY

-WEAR A LOVE-GLOVE

-TAKE A SHOWER

-GET A HAIRCUT

-ASK HER OUT

-OPEN WITH A JOKE

-DON'T BE CREEPY

-WEAR A LOVE-GLOVE

-TAKE A SHOWER

-GET A HAIRCUT

-ASK HER OUT

-OPEN WITH A JOKE

-DON'T BE CREEPY

-WEAR A LOVE-GLOVE

-TAKE A SHOWER

-GET A HAIRCUT

-ASK HER OUT

-OPEN WITH A JOKE

-DON'T BE CREEPY

-WEAR A LOVE-GLOVE

THE END

R J DUNCAN MAKES HIS LIVING WRITING SILLY BOOKS LIKE THIS ONE AND MAYBE SOMETHING A BIT MORE SERIOUS FROM TIME TO TIME. IF YOU ENJOYED THIS BOOK, CHECK OUT ALL THE OTHER ONES,

OR

IF YOU WOULD LIKE DUNCAN TO MAKE A BOOK JUST FOR YOU, WITH YOU PICKING ALL OF THE CONTENT, GET IN TOUCH:

www.RJDUNCANBOOKS.com

BECAUSE WHO THE HELL DOESN'T WANT A BOOK MADE FOR THEIR BIRTHDAY, BACHELOR'S PARTY, FAMILY GATHERING, FLAG DAY?